The Ampicillin Handbook

Understanding Usage and How This Essential Antibiotic Fights Infection Safely and Effectively

Daisy Farr

Copyright

© **2025 Daisy Farr**. All rights reserved.

No part of this publication may be reproduced, distributed, or transmitted in any form or by any means, including photocopying, recording, or other electronic or mechanical methods, without the prior written permission of the author, except in the case of brief quotations embodied in critical reviews or scholarly articles.

Disclaimer:

This guide is intended for informational purposes only and is not a substitute for professional medical advice, diagnosis, or treatment. Always seek the advice of your physician or other qualified healthcare provider with any questions you may have regarding a medical condition or medication.

The author and publisher disclaim any liability for any injury, illness, or damages arising from the use or misuse of the information contained within this guide. Treatment decisions should always be made in consultation with a licensed healthcare professional.

Table of Contents

Getting to Know Ampicillin	4
How Ampicillin Works in the Body	8
Medical Conditions Treated with Ampicillin	14
Proper Use and Dosing Guidelines	22
Potential Side Effects and Safety Profile	29
Warnings, Interactions, and When to Avoid Use	37
Antibiotic Resistance and Effectiveness in Modern Practice	46
Using Ampicillin Safely: Practical Advice for Patients	54

Getting to Know Ampicillin

Ampicillin is a well-established and widely used antibiotic that has been a mainstay in the treatment of bacterial infections since the 1960s. As part of the penicillin family, it works by targeting the walls of bacteria, ultimately stopping their growth and helping your immune system eliminate the infection. Despite the introduction of many newer antibiotics, ampicillin remains a trusted treatment option for a range of infections due to its proven effectiveness, affordability, and safety record.

Ampicillin is classified as a **broad-spectrum antibiotic**, which means it can act against both

Gram-positive and some Gram-negative bacteria. This versatility allows it to be used for various infections, including respiratory tract infections, urinary tract infections (UTIs), gastrointestinal infections, and certain forms of meningitis. It's also commonly used in both adult and pediatric care settings.

One of the key benefits of ampicillin is that it can be taken orally or given through an injection, offering flexibility depending on the severity of the infection and the needs of the patient. In hospitals, intravenous (IV) ampicillin is often used for more serious conditions, while oral capsules or suspensions are typical for outpatient treatment.

Like many antibiotics, ampicillin is only effective against **bacterial** infections—not viruses like the flu or the common cold. This distinction is essential to avoid unnecessary use, which contributes to the growing global problem of antibiotic resistance. Responsible prescribing and proper use of ampicillin help preserve its effectiveness for future patients.

In most cases, ampicillin is well tolerated when used correctly. However, as with any medication, there are considerations to be aware of, including allergic reactions (particularly in people with penicillin allergies), interactions with other drugs, and side effects that will be covered in later chapters.

Understanding how and when to use ampicillin is the first step in ensuring safe, effective treatment. This guide is designed to equip you with the knowledge to navigate your antibiotic treatment confidently and responsibly—whether you're a patient, caregiver, or simply someone seeking to make more informed health decisions.

How Ampicillin Works in the Body

Ampicillin is a member of the beta-lactam class of antibiotics, which includes penicillin and its derivatives. These antibiotics are effective because they interfere with a critical function of bacterial survival: the construction of their cell walls.

Bacteria, unlike human cells, have rigid outer cell walls made of a substance called peptidoglycan. This wall helps maintain the shape of the bacteria and protects them from environmental stress. Ampicillin works by blocking the enzymes (called penicillin-binding proteins, or PBPs) that bacteria need to build and maintain this cell wall.

When ampicillin enters the bacterial environment, it binds to these PBPs and disrupts the wall-building process. This leads to weakened cell walls and eventually causes the bacteria to rupture and die—a process known as bactericidal activity.

Absorption and Distribution

When taken orally, ampicillin is absorbed through the digestive tract and enters the bloodstream. Its absorption, however, can be reduced if taken with food, so it's usually recommended on an empty stomach for optimal effectiveness.

Once in the bloodstream, ampicillin distributes throughout the body, including into the lungs, bile, and urinary tract. It can also cross into the cerebrospinal fluid when the brain's protective barrier becomes inflamed, such as during meningitis. This broad distribution makes it useful for treating a wide range of infections.

Elimination from the Body

Ampicillin is primarily removed from the body by the kidneys, meaning that it is excreted in the urine. This characteristic makes it especially effective for urinary tract infections, as high concentrations can be achieved in the urinary system.

In patients with reduced kidney function, the drug may take longer to clear from the body, and dosing adjustments are often necessary to avoid accumulation and toxicity.

Spectrum of Activity

Ampicillin is classified as a broad-spectrum antibiotic, which means it targets a wider range of bacteria compared to earlier penicillins. Specifically, it works against many Gram-positive organisms (such as *Streptococcus pneumoniae* and *Enterococcus faecalis*) and some Gram-negative bacteria (such as *Escherichia coli*, *Haemophilus influenzae*, and *Salmonella* species).

However, some bacteria have developed ways to resist ampicillin's effects. One of the most common resistance mechanisms is the production of beta-lactamase—an enzyme that breaks down the beta-lactam ring in ampicillin, rendering it ineffective. To counter this, ampicillin is sometimes combined with beta-lactamase inhibitors such as sulbactam.

In simple terms, ampicillin works by disrupting bacterial cell wall production, leading to bacterial death. Its ability to reach various parts of the body and its effectiveness against a broad range of bacteria make it a valuable tool in treating infections. Understanding how it works helps ensure it's used properly—maximizing benefits while minimizing risks like resistance or side effects.

Medical Conditions Treated with Ampicillin

Ampicillin is widely used in clinical medicine due to its ability to treat a broad range of bacterial infections. As a broad-spectrum penicillin antibiotic, it is effective against many Gram-positive and some Gram-negative organisms. Its versatility makes it suitable for treating infections in both outpatient and hospital settings.

Below are some of the most common medical conditions for which ampicillin is prescribed.

1. Respiratory Tract Infections

Ampicillin is often used to treat upper and lower respiratory tract infections caused by susceptible bacteria. These include:

- **Pharyngitis** (throat infections)

- **Tonsillitis**

- **Bronchitis**

- **Pneumonia**

In cases where the infection is caused by *Streptococcus pneumoniae* or *Haemophilus influenzae*, ampicillin can be an effective first-line treatment. It is particularly useful when sensitivity to the drug has been confirmed through laboratory testing.

2. Urinary Tract Infections (UTIs)

Due to its renal elimination, ampicillin reaches high concentrations in the urinary tract, making it effective for treating UTIs caused by bacteria such as:

- *Escherichia coli*

- *Enterococcus faecalis*

- *Proteus mirabilis*

UTIs are among the most frequent reasons for outpatient antibiotic prescriptions, and ampicillin remains an option when the causative organism is known to be sensitive.

3. Gastrointestinal Infections

Ampicillin can be used to treat certain gastrointestinal infections, including:

- **Typhoid fever** (caused by *Salmonella typhi*)

- **Shigellosis** (caused by *Shigella* species)

- **Listeriosis** (caused by *Listeria monocytogenes*)

In the case of **Listeria**, ampicillin is often used in combination with other antibiotics such as gentamicin for a synergistic effect.

4. Meningitis

Ampicillin plays a critical role in the treatment of bacterial meningitis, especially when caused by:

- *Listeria monocytogenes*

- Group B *Streptococcus*

- *Enterococcus* species

In newborns, the elderly, and immunocompromised patients, Listeria is a concern, and ampicillin is frequently included in empiric treatment regimens.

5. Endocarditis

Ampicillin is also used in the treatment of bacterial endocarditis, particularly infections caused by enterococci. In these cases, it is commonly administered intravenously and often combined with aminoglycosides like gentamicin to improve bacterial clearance from heart tissue.

6. Gynecological and Obstetric Infections

In obstetric settings, ampicillin may be used to treat:

- Chorioamnionitis

- Postpartum infections

- Group B Streptococcus (GBS) prophylaxis during labor for women who test positive for GBS colonization

Its use in these scenarios helps prevent serious infections in both mothers and newborns.

7. Sepsis and Systemic Infections

For serious systemic infections, especially in infants and immunocompromised patients, ampicillin can be a key part of empiric therapy—treatment given before the exact cause of infection is known. Its spectrum and safety profile make it a valuable choice in these high-risk situations.

Proper Use and Dosing Guidelines

Ampicillin is most effective when used as directed and tailored to the type and severity of the infection being treated. Correct dosing ensures that therapeutic levels are reached in the body, which helps eliminate the infection while minimizing side effects and the risk of bacterial resistance.

General Principles of Use

Ampicillin is available in several forms:

- **Oral capsules**

- **Oral suspension (liquid)**

- **Intravenous (IV) or intramuscular (IM) injections**

The route of administration depends on the infection's location and severity. Oral forms are typically used for mild to moderate infections, while IV or IM forms are used in hospital settings for serious or systemic infections.

It is essential to **complete the full course** of ampicillin, even if symptoms improve early. Stopping treatment too soon can allow the infection to return and may contribute to antibiotic resistance.

Timing and Food Considerations

Oral ampicillin should be taken **on an empty stomach**, ideally **30 to 60 minutes before a meal** or **2 hours after eating**, because food can interfere with its absorption in the gastrointestinal tract. Always take it with a full glass of water, unless otherwise directed.

For patients using the oral suspension, the bottle should be **shaken well** before each use to ensure even distribution of the medication.

Typical Dosing Guidelines

The appropriate dosage of ampicillin varies by **age, weight, kidney function, and the type of infection**. Below are common dosing examples for different populations and conditions. All dosages should be confirmed by a healthcare provider.

1. Adults

- **Uncomplicated respiratory or urinary infections**: 250–500 mg every 6 hours

- **Severe infections or systemic infections**: Up to 1–2 g every 4–6 hours IV

- **Listeria meningitis**: Often 2 g IV every 4 hours, combined with gentamicin

2. Children

- Dosing is usually **based on body weight** (mg/kg)

- **Mild to moderate infections**: 50–100 mg/kg/day divided every 6 hours

- **Serious infections**: 100–200 mg/kg/day, or more, depending on severity

3. Newborns and Infants

    - Dosages are carefully adjusted based on age (in days or weeks) and weight

    - Used commonly in neonatal sepsis and meningitis

4. Pregnant or Breastfeeding Individuals

Ampicillin is considered relatively safe during pregnancy and breastfeeding. However, dosing may be adjusted based on physiological changes during pregnancy. It is also used as part of **Group B Streptococcus (GBS)** prophylaxis during labor.

Kidney Function and Dose Adjustment

Since ampicillin is eliminated primarily by the kidneys, patients with **impaired renal function** may require dose adjustments to prevent drug accumulation. Healthcare providers often order lab tests (such as creatinine clearance) to determine appropriate dosing in these cases.

Missed Doses and Overdose

If a dose is missed, it should be taken as soon as remembered. If it's close to the next scheduled dose, skip the missed one—**do not double up**. In case of accidental overdose, symptoms may include severe nausea, vomiting, or signs of allergic reaction. Immediate medical attention should be sought.

Potential Side Effects and Safety Profile

Like all medications, ampicillin can cause side effects. While most people tolerate it well, being aware of possible reactions allows patients and healthcare providers to respond quickly and appropriately if problems arise.

Common Side Effects

Most of the common side effects of ampicillin are mild and temporary. These include:

- **Gastrointestinal disturbances**: Nausea, vomiting, diarrhea, and abdominal discomfort are among the most frequently reported issues. These symptoms are usually mild and resolve without intervention. Taking the medication with a full glass of water and on an empty stomach may help reduce stomach upset.

- **Skin rash**:

    A non-serious rash may appear, especially in children or those being treated for viral infections like mononucleosis. This rash is typically flat, red, and not itchy. However, a rash should always be reported to a healthcare provider to rule out a more serious allergic reaction.

Allergic Reactions

Ampicillin, like other penicillins, can trigger allergic reactions in sensitive individuals. These reactions can vary in severity:

- **Mild allergic reactions** may include:

  - Itching

  - Hives

  - Mild swelling

- **Severe allergic reactions (anaphylaxis)** are rare but require immediate medical attention. Symptoms include:

- Difficulty breathing

- Swelling of the face, lips, tongue, or throat

- Rapid heartbeat

- Dizziness or fainting

Patients with a known allergy to penicillin or any beta-lactam antibiotic should not take ampicillin unless under strict medical supervision.

Superinfection Risk

In some cases, prolonged use of antibiotics like ampicillin can lead to the overgrowth of non-susceptible organisms, such as fungi or resistant bacteria. This is called a superinfection. One common example is oral or vaginal yeast infections caused by *Candida* species.

In rare cases, a more serious complication called Clostridioides difficile–associated diarrhea (CDAD) may occur. This condition causes severe, persistent diarrhea and requires specialized treatment.

Effects on Blood and Liver

Infrequently, ampicillin may affect blood cells or liver function. These effects are more common with prolonged or high-dose use and typically resolve after the drug is discontinued.

Possible effects include:

- **Mild elevations in liver enzymes**

- **Anemia or low white blood cell count**

- **Eosinophilia** (a type of elevated white blood cell count often linked to allergic reactions)

Routine blood tests are not usually needed for short-term treatment but may be monitored in patients receiving prolonged therapy or those with underlying health conditions.

Use in Special Populations

- **Children**: Ampicillin is commonly used and generally well-tolerated in children, but dosing must be carefully adjusted by weight.

- **Pregnant individuals**: Considered relatively safe during pregnancy, and often used for specific indications such as Group B Streptococcus prophylaxis during labor.

- **Older adults**: May be more sensitive to gastrointestinal side effects and may require dose adjustment if kidney function is reduced.

When to Seek Medical Advice

Patients should contact a healthcare provider immediately if they experience:

- Persistent or severe diarrhea

- Signs of allergic reaction

- Unusual fatigue or bruising

- Yellowing of the skin or eyes (jaundice)

Warnings, Interactions, and When to Avoid Use

Although ampicillin is a widely used and generally safe antibiotic, certain individuals should avoid it, and others should use it with caution. Understanding the drug's warnings, potential interactions, and contraindications is essential to ensure safe and effective use.

When Ampicillin Should Be Avoided

Ampicillin should **not** be used in the following circumstances:

- **Known Allergy to Penicillins**: Anyone with a history of allergic reactions—mild or severe—to penicillin or other beta-lactam antibiotics (such as amoxicillin or cephalosporins) should avoid ampicillin unless there is no suitable alternative and close medical supervision is available.

- **Hypersensitivity Reactions**:

  Past episodes of serious skin rashes, breathing difficulties, or anaphylaxis following antibiotic use are absolute reasons to avoid ampicillin.

- **Mononucleosis (Epstein-Barr Virus Infection)**:

  Ampicillin is known to cause a widespread rash in patients with mononucleosis. Though not dangerous, the rash can be mistaken for a drug allergy and should therefore be avoided in these cases.

Drug Interactions

Like all medications, ampicillin can interact with other drugs. Some interactions may reduce its effectiveness, while others may increase the risk of side effects.

Here are some key interactions to be aware of:

- **Oral Contraceptives**: There is limited but notable evidence that ampicillin may reduce the effectiveness of birth control pills. While this interaction remains controversial, it is often recommended to use **backup contraception** during antibiotic therapy.

- **Allopurinol**:

    Taking allopurinol (used to treat gout) alongside ampicillin increases the risk of skin rashes. This combination should be avoided if possible.

- **Anticoagulants (e.g., warfarin)**:

    Ampicillin may enhance the effects of anticoagulants, potentially increasing the risk of bleeding. Regular monitoring of clotting levels may be needed if both drugs are used together.

- **Other Antibiotics**:

    Using ampicillin with bacteriostatic

antibiotics like tetracyclines may reduce its effectiveness. These drugs work in different ways, and their actions may interfere with one another.

- **Methotrexate**:
  Ampicillin can decrease the clearance of methotrexate, a medication used for cancer and autoimmune diseases, leading to increased toxicity. Dose adjustments or close monitoring may be necessary.

Use with Caution

Certain individuals can use ampicillin, but only under medical guidance:

- **Patients with Renal Impairment**:
  Ampicillin is primarily eliminated by the kidneys. In people with impaired kidney function, the drug can accumulate to harmful levels if the dose is not adjusted appropriately.

- **Pregnant and Breastfeeding Individuals**:
  Ampicillin is generally considered safe during pregnancy and lactation, but healthcare providers should always assess risks versus benefits.

- **People with a History of Seizures**:
  Although rare, high doses of ampicillin—particularly in individuals with kidney disease or pre-existing

seizure disorders—may increase the risk of seizures.

- **Newborns and Premature Infants**:

  Dosing must be carefully calculated by weight and kidney function. Neonates eliminate the drug more slowly, so lower doses or longer intervals between doses are often required.

Food and Absorption

Ampicillin's effectiveness can be reduced if taken with food. To optimize absorption, it should be taken **on an empty stomach**, ideally **1 hour before or 2 hours after meals**.

Laboratory Monitoring

While routine monitoring isn't necessary for short-term, low-dose use, long-term or high-dose use—especially in hospital settings—may require:

- **Kidney function tests**

- **Liver enzyme monitoring**

- **Blood cell counts**

Antibiotic Resistance and Effectiveness in Modern Practice

Ampicillin has played a pivotal role in antibiotic therapy since its introduction in the 1960s. However, like all antibiotics, its effectiveness is being challenged by the global rise in bacterial resistance. Understanding how resistance develops, where ampicillin still works well, and how research is responding is essential to ensure its continued clinical value.

Ampicillin's Legacy of Effectiveness

Ampicillin is a broad-spectrum beta-lactam antibiotic. It remains effective against a wide range of **Gram-positive** organisms (such as *Streptococcus pneumoniae* and *Enterococcus faecalis*) and many **Gram-negative** bacteria (like *Haemophilus influenzae* and *Escherichia coli*).

In clinical practice today, ampicillin is still widely used for:

- **Pediatric respiratory infections**

- **Meningitis caused by *Listeria monocytogenes***

- **Urinary tract infections (UTIs)**

- **Group B Streptococcus prophylaxis during childbirth**

- **Severe enterococcal infections (often with gentamicin)**

However, its role has narrowed due to rising resistance and the availability of newer antibiotics with broader coverage.

The Rise of Resistance

Over time, many bacteria have developed the ability to resist ampicillin's effects, largely due to:

- **Beta-lactamase production**: Some bacteria produce enzymes called beta-lactamases that break down the antibiotic before it can act. This is one of the most common mechanisms of resistance against ampicillin.

- **Genetic mutations**:

   Changes in the structure of bacterial cell walls or penicillin-binding proteins can reduce the drug's ability to attach and work effectively.

- **Efflux pumps and reduced permeability**:

   Bacteria may develop systems to pump out the drug or prevent it from entering their cells.

Resistance is particularly common among:

- **Enterobacteriaceae (e.g., *E. coli*, *Klebsiella*)**

- **Beta-lactamase–producing** *Haemophilus influenzae*

- **Some strains of** *Neisseria gonorrhoeae*

- **Hospital-acquired infections**, where antibiotic exposure is frequent

Combating Resistance

One strategy to preserve ampicillin's usefulness is combining it with a **beta-lactamase inhibitor**, such as **sulbactam**. These combinations can extend the drug's spectrum by neutralizing the enzymes that destroy it.

In addition, healthcare systems are working to:

- Promote **antibiotic stewardship**, ensuring ampicillin is only used when appropriate

- Develop better **diagnostic tools** to guide targeted therapy

- Encourage **shorter courses** of therapy when evidence supports it, reducing selection pressure on bacteria

Current Research and Innovation

Ongoing research into ampicillin and beta-lactam antibiotics focuses on several key areas:

- **Understanding resistance mechanisms** at the molecular level to design more robust drugs

- **Monitoring global resistance patterns** to update treatment guidelines

- **Developing new beta-lactamase inhibitors** to pair with older antibiotics

- **Improving delivery methods**, such as sustained-release formulations or targeted IV infusions

In some infections—especially those in **low-resource settings**—ampicillin remains the drug of choice because of its **affordability, availability, and clinical familiarity**. In hospital environments, it continues to play a critical role in treating specific serious infections when susceptibility is confirmed.

Using Ampicillin Safely: Practical Advice for Patients

Ampicillin is a valuable antibiotic that has helped millions recover from bacterial infections. To get the best results and stay safe during treatment, it's important to follow practical advice and understand how to use this medication correctly.

Follow Your Prescription Exactly

- **Take the full course:** Even if you start feeling better, complete the entire prescribed course of ampicillin. Stopping early can allow bacteria to survive, leading to a return of infection or antibiotic resistance.

- **Stick to the schedule:** Take ampicillin at the times prescribed, usually every 6 to 8 hours, depending on your dose. Setting alarms or using pill organizers can help you remember.

- **Do not skip doses:** Missing doses can reduce the medicine's effectiveness. If you do miss a dose, take it as soon as you remember unless it's nearly time for your next dose. Never double up.

How to Take Ampicillin

- **Take on an empty stomach:** Ampicillin is best absorbed when taken 1 hour before or 2 hours after meals. Drinking a full glass of water with each dose helps the medicine dissolve and reach your bloodstream efficiently.

- **For liquid forms:** Shake the bottle well before measuring a dose. Use a proper measuring spoon or cup—not household teaspoons—to ensure accurate dosing.

Watch for Side Effects

- Mild side effects such as nausea, diarrhea, or mild rash are common. If these become severe or persistent, contact your healthcare provider.

- If you experience any signs of an allergic reaction—such as rash, itching, swelling, or difficulty breathing—seek emergency medical care immediately.

Avoid Unnecessary Interactions

- **Inform your healthcare provider** about all medications, vitamins, or supplements you are taking to avoid interactions.

- Use alternative contraception methods during treatment if you rely on hormonal birth control, as antibiotics can sometimes reduce their effectiveness.

- Avoid alcohol during antibiotic therapy as it may increase side effects like stomach upset or dizziness.

Special Considerations

- **Kidney health:** If you have kidney problems, your doctor may adjust your dose. Always inform them about any existing kidney issues.

- **Pregnancy and breastfeeding:** Ampicillin is generally safe, but always consult your doctor before use.

- **Storage:** Keep ampicillin capsules and liquids in a cool, dry place away from direct sunlight. For the oral suspension, refrigeration is often recommended—check the label for specific instructions.

When to Contact Your Healthcare Provider

- If symptoms persist or worsen despite treatment

- If you develop severe diarrhea, which could indicate *Clostridioides difficile* infection

- Any new or unusual symptoms during therapy

- Questions or concerns about medication use

By following these practical steps, patients can maximize the effectiveness of ampicillin treatment while minimizing risks. Always maintain open communication with your healthcare team, and never hesitate to ask questions about your medication.

About the Author

Daisy Farr is a dedicated healthcare writer and medical educator with a passion for making complex medical information accessible to everyone. With a background in pharmacology and years of experience working alongside healthcare professionals, Daisy brings clarity and insight to topics related to antibiotics and infectious diseases.

Her mission is to empower patients and practitioners alike with trustworthy, up-to-date knowledge that supports safe and effective treatment decisions. When not writing, Daisy enjoys volunteering in community health programs and advocating for patient education.

Through her work, Daisy Farr continues to contribute to better health outcomes by bridging the gap between medical science and everyday understanding.

Made in the USA
Middletown, DE
27 June 2025

77595988R00035